Myelody Syndrom

GH00976236

Contents

© Ian Banks 2009. Date for revision: 2011

Cartoons by Jim Campbell. All photos © istockphoto.com.

ISBN: 978 1 906121 84 6

(021-12420)

Printed in the UK.

Haynes Publishing, Sparkford, Yeovil, Somerset BA22 7JJ, England

Haynes North America, Inc, 861 Lawrence Drive, Newbury Park, California 91320, USA

Haynes Publishing Nordiska AB, Box 1504, 751 45 Uppsala, Sweden

The Author and the Publisher have taken care to ensure that the advice given in this edition is current at the time of publication. The Reader is advised to read and understand the instructions and information material included with all medicines recommended, and to consider carefully the appropriateness of any treatments. The Author and the Publisher will have no liability for adverse results, inappropriate or excessive use of the remedies offered in this book or their level of effectiveness in individual cases. The Author and the Publisher do not intend that this book be used as a substitute for medical advice. Advice from a medical practitioner should always be sought for any symptom or illness.

Introduction

What are Myelodysplastic Syndromes (MDS)?

So, let's get the basics sorted before we talk about treatment. Myelodysplastic syndromes (MDS) are a group of diseases that affect the blood cell production in the bone marrow. They are not all the same, some types of MDS are mild and easily managed, while other types are severe and life-threatening. Thankfully, while there is not always a cure, they can all be treated at the very least to slow disease progression and reduce tiredness.

It is a mixture of good and bad news, mild MDS can grow more severe over time. It can also develop into a fast-growing, severe leukaemia called acute myelogenous leukaemia (AML). This is not inevitable and can still be treated.

The best treatment for a person with MDS depends on his or her type of MDS, risk level, age, overall health and his or her own preferences. The treatment options include:

- Supportive care.
- Bone marrow or cord blood transplant (BMT).
- Chemotherapy.
- Newer therapy options.

If you are diagnosed with MDS, it is important to talk with a doctor who has experience treating MDS. Don't be afraid to ask about this. Doctors are very used to being asked about their medical experience.

Ask about the type of MDS you have, your risk factors and treatment options, and discuss your own treatment goals. There are a variety of treatment options available, including newer treatments being studied in clinical trials. Give yourself time to think and consider. Write things down, ask for written information about the hospital unit which will be looking after you. Don't make your decision straight away. Talk to your partner, relatives and friends. You have time to get it right for you.

What do you want to know about MDS?

We have a truly amazing medical profession but sometimes it can tend to speak rather than listen. The most important person in the room is you and you need answers to questions which can often be difficult to ask. This manual will give you some of the answers but more importantly make it easier for you to talk about your medical condition with health professionals and other people who care about you. Making decisions over treatment options is not always straightforward or easy. Understanding the pros and cons, the plus and minus of different treatments can help guide you to what you want from modern treatments. Hopefully this manual will supply most of the answers but it cannot take the place of talking to your doctor or nurse.

Is MDS inheritable?

Although a genetic change is linked to MDS there is no evidence that it can be inherited from either the male or female parent.

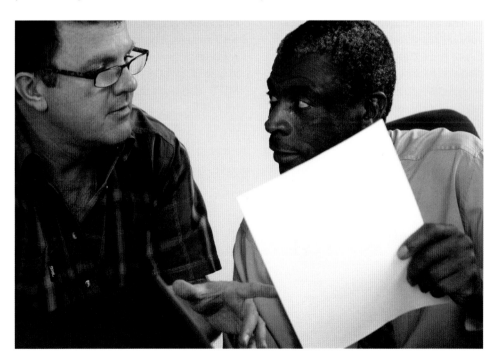

I have never heard of MDS

Is it a new disease?

No, but it took a while to sort out all the different symptoms. Since the early 20th century it began to be recognised that some people with acute myelogenous leukaemia had a preceding period of anaemia and abnormal blood cell production. These conditions were lumped with other diseases under the term 'refractory anaemia'. The first description of 'pre-leukaemia' as a specific entity was published in 1953 and the syndrome went by many names until 1976 when the term MDS was popularised.

The likely course of MDS can be very different for different people. Experience has shown that certain disease factors affect a person's prognosis – his or her chances of long-term survival and risk of developing AML. Researchers use these factors to classify MDS into types (also see *Risk scores* on page 31).

The two more common types of MDS are refractory anaemia (RA) and refractory anaemia with ringed sideroblasts (RARS). These are also the less severe forms of MDS. They have a lower risk of turning into AML. Some patients with these forms of MDS may live with few symptoms and need little treatment for many years.

The other types of MDS tend to be more severe and more difficult to treat successfully. The refractory anaemia with excess blasts (RAEB) and refractory anaemia with excess blasts in transformation (RAEB-t) forms of MDS also have a higher risk of turning into AML.

What causes MDS?

As with many medical conditions, there are more questions than answers when it comes to what causes them. In MDS, the bone marrow does not make enough normal blood cells for the body. One, two or all three types of blood cells – red blood cells, white blood cells and platelets – may be affected. The marrow may also make unformed cells called blasts.

Blasts normally develop into red blood cells, white blood cells or platelets. In MDS, the blasts are abnormal and do not develop or function normally.

Most often the cause of the changes to the bone marrow is unknown. This is called de novo MDS. In a small number of people, MDS might be linked to heavy exposure to some chemicals, such as certain solvents or pesticides, or to radiation. MDS can also be caused by treatment for other diseases. This is called treatment-related MDS or secondary MDS. It can be helpful to write down any possible exposure you might have had to the risk factors above to identify a possible secondary MDS.

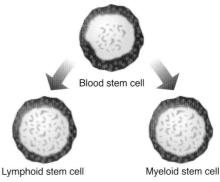

Blood stem cell

Lymphoid stem cell   Myeloid stem cell

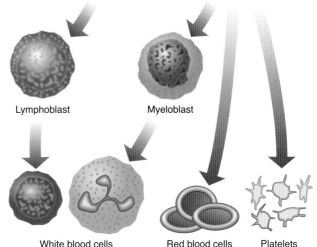

Lymphoblast   Myeloblast

White blood cells   Red blood cells   Platelets

How common is MDS?

MDS is relatively rare, with an incidence estimated at up to 50 cases per 100,000 people per year. Although MDS can affect people of any age, more than 80% of cases are in people over age 60. MDS is more common in men than in women.

Why didn't my GP diagnose my MDS earlier?

Most of the older patients don't go to see their doctor because they are thinking the symptoms are normal; being exhausted and tired are normal results for their age. Unfortunately the often vague symptoms of MDS can mimic other medical conditions, especially when they are mild. Tiredness, a common symptom, can be put down to over-work, stress, poor sleep and so on. Worse still, the symptoms also depend on the severity of the disease. Many people with MDS have no symptoms when they are diagnosed. Their disease is found through a routine blood test. If a person does have symptoms, they are usually caused by low numbers of blood cells. Classically it will be tiredness from anaemia, a common symptom in itself.

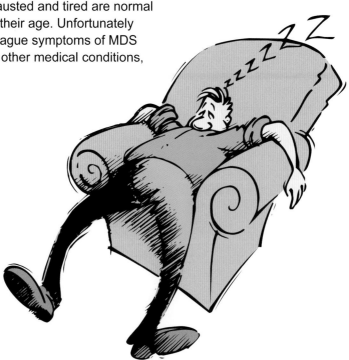

Is the poor awareness because MDS affects old people?

It is true that although MDS can affect people of any age, more than 80% of cases are in people over 60. We know that older people do tend to come off worse in many ways in our society, which appears to value youth more than experience and wisdom. In fairness, MDS is a group of diseases with symptoms that are often treated without the doctor finding their cause.

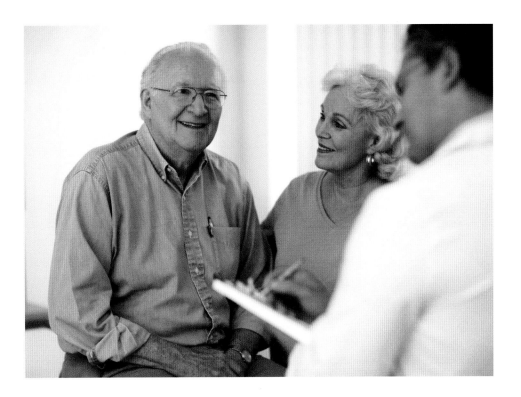

What are the symptoms of MDS?

There are several different sorts of blood cell. The symptoms of MDS can vary depending on which types of cells are affected. The common symptoms are as follows:

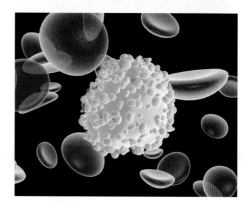

- Low numbers of red blood cells can lead to anaemia with feeling tired or weak, being short of breath and looking pale. Anaemia is the most common symptom of MDS.

- Low numbers of white blood cells can lead to fever and frequent infections.

- Low numbers of platelets can lead to easy bleeding or bruising.

- Weight loss.

In severe MDS, infection or uncontrolled bleeding can be dangerous.

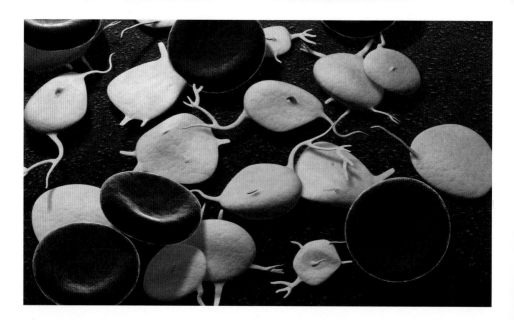

Are the doctors sure I have MDS?

Other people have different symptoms

MDS has many and different symptoms. Doctors look at samples of blood and bone marrow to diagnose MDS. They also look for changes in the chromosomes (the genetic material inside the cells) of bone marrow cells (cytogenetics).

MDS can sometimes be hard to diagnose. Careful study of blood and marrow samples is needed to tell MDS apart from other diseases with similar signs and symptoms, such as anaemia from other causes (eg, aplastic anaemia). Blood and marrow samples are often tested several times over two or more months to find out whether the disease is stable or getting worse.

It is important to diagnose the type of MDS to make the best treatment choices. With some types of MDS, a person may live with few symptoms for years, while other types can be life-threatening within months. In addition, some types of MDS are more likely than others to develop into acute myelogenous leukaemia (AML). Yes, AML that develops from MDS can be hard to treat, but the main thing to remember is that treatment is out there and getting better all the time.

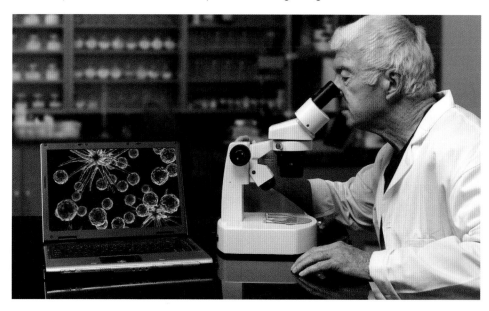

I have MDS

What can I do to keep myself healthy?

Good question, not least because it opens the door to what you can do to help take control of the situation Because people with certain myelodysplastic syndromes have low white cell counts, they're subject to recurrent, and often serious, infections. The chemotherapy which is sometimes used to treat the most severe forms of MDS, either on its own or before a stem cell transplant, increases the risk. Experts recommend the following measures to help reduce the chance of infection:

● Protect the neck and chest with a scarf to avoid a cold.

● Wash your hands. Frequent hand washing is the best way to control infection especially from flu which is mainly from physical contact. Wash your hands thoroughly with warm, soapy water, especially before eating or preparing food. Carry an alcohol-based hand rub for times when water isn't available.

● Take care with food. Thoroughly cook all meat and fish. Avoid fruits and vegetables that you can't peel, especially lettuce, and wash all produce you do use before peeling. To be absolutely safe, you may want to avoid raw foods entirely.

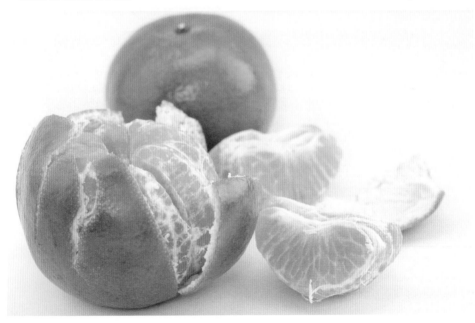

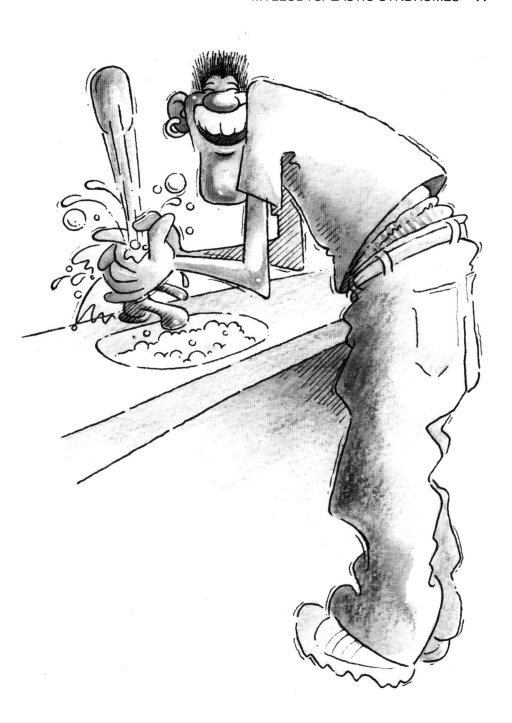

- Avoid people who are ill, especially with chickenpox and shingles.

Myelodysplastic syndromes can affect your immune system.

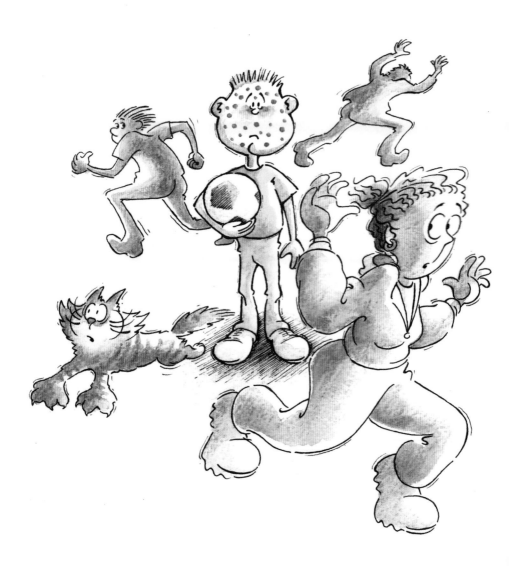

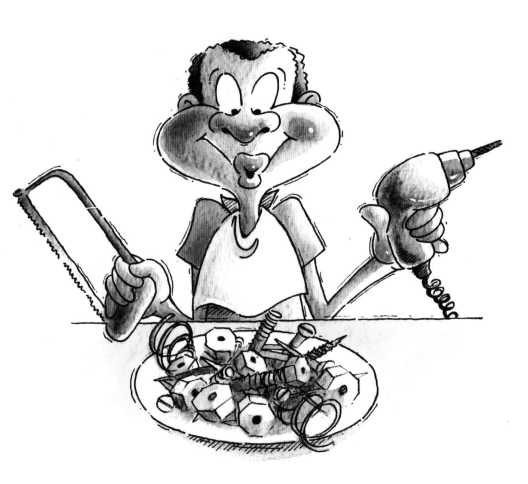

Should I follow a diet rich in iron?

The short answer is no, unless your doctor advises you to; there is no need to take multi-vitamins with added iron, either. Iron is very poorly absorbed from the gut. If you have been receiving blood transfusions chances are you will have too much rather than too little iron on board. Tiredness and exhaustion is more related to the number of red blood cells rather the amount of iron.

Are there changes to make in my daily life?

I get very tired – what can I do to get more energy?

With MDS, you may find your interest in your normal activities declines. Activities you used to enjoy may become a burden, tire you out, or simply not interest you any more. Discuss your feelings openly with your friends, relatives and doctors. There are many possible ways to rekindle your interest in life. There are also medications that might help. Other general recommendations that may help include:

- Follow a nutritious diet.
- Participate in a reasonable level of exercise.
- Rest when tired.

Eating a healthy diet may help you avoid other medical conditions linked to poor nutrition. Because MDS itself and some MDS treatments may have a dulling effect on your appetite, it's important that you make the most of the calories you do take in. Avoid making drastic changes in your food based on the latest fad diet.

It's important that you don't make

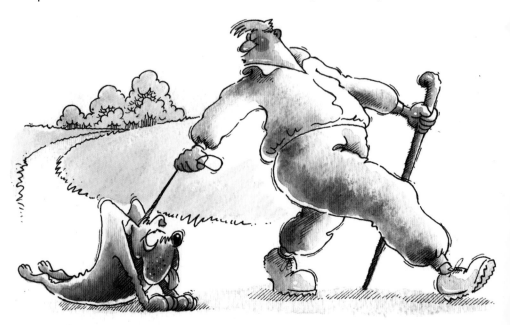

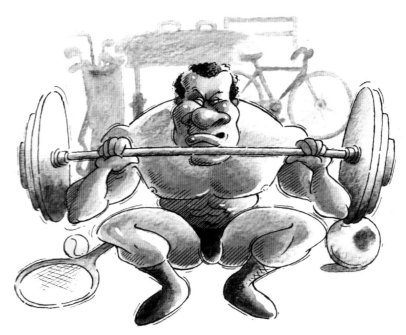

major lifestyle changes without consulting your doctor and checking that you are doing things safely. You are already being physically and emotionally challenged by your MDS and the rigors of treatment. You and your doctor need to work together to make wise lifestyle choices and implement them in the healthiest way possible.

If you have not been exercising regularly, check with your doctor to determine a safe exercise program which suits you best. Exercise has many benefits that may help you withstand the physical and emotional stresses of MDS and its treatment:

● Promoting overall fitness.

● Boosting your energy level.

● Improving the functioning of your immune system.

● Bolstering your spirits and improving your emotional outlook.

Think about joining a gym to help you set exercise goals and to safely follow through on starting up an exercise program.

Be sure to balance rest and activities to prevent becoming too tired.

The treatments for MDS can add to the fatigue you already feel from fighting MDS. In fact, fatigue is the most frequently experienced symptom of MDS and MDS treatments. The fatigue you feel can range from 'just feeling tired' to complete and utter exhaustion. Wherever in this range you fall, you may find your tiredness quite distressing and affecting your quality of life.

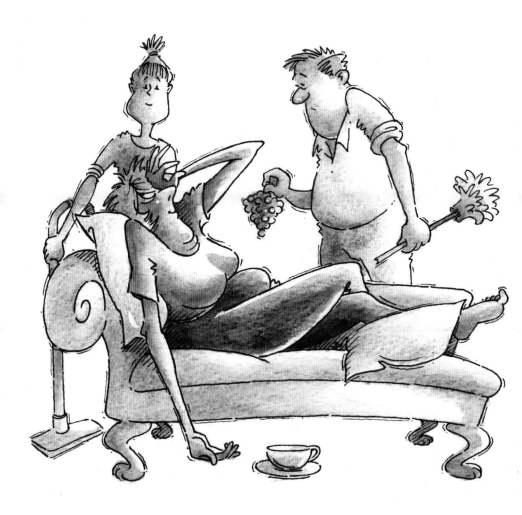

So, to help avoid getting overtired, try not to do too much. Prioritise the things you need to do, and focus on the most important ones. Also, allow others to help you with daily chores, shopping, and preparing meals. Plan times throughout the day when you can rest.

Is it safe to exercise with low haemoglobin?

Haemoglobin is the iron-containing protein found in red blood cells that carries oxygen. A lack of it or of the red blood cells themselves causes anaemia, which can make you very tired, exhausted even, making any sort of activity difficult. On the other hand, exercise is good for the body's defence system and general well being, not least your morale. Pushing yourself too hard can be dangerous as there is less oxygen going to the heart and brain. This can cause a very fast heart rate or fainting, especially when standing up quickly after too much exercise. Fainting is not serious in itself but can cause injury as a result of the fall. A reasonable rule of thumb is to stop activity for a while if it is making you breathless or dizzy. Don't try to 'walk through the barrier' like joggers in a marathon. Sit down, or even better, lie down with your feet on a pillow, until your breathing returns to normal. Your doctor will know your level of anaemia and can advise you.

There are support services that can make activity (such as using the stairs) much easier and less tiring. Even a stick, walking frame or perch stool can make simple tasks like cooking or making tea or coffee possible and safer. Ask your doctor or social worker.

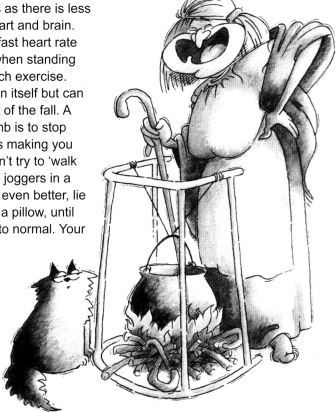

What precautions should I take to avoid infection?

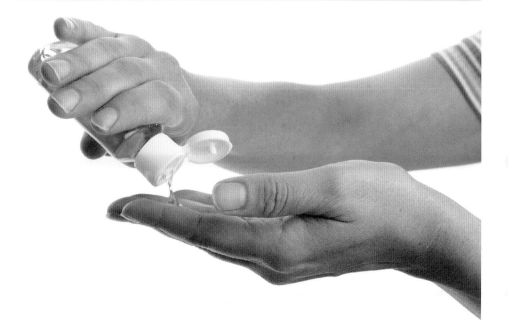

A lower than normal number of white blood cells can leave you open to infections. There are some commonsense things you can do to decrease your risk of infection and avoid exposure to bacteria and viruses:

- Try to avoid crowds, especially during the cold and flu season.
- Ask your doctor about immunisation against the flu and pneumonia.
- Wash your hands thoroughly and often. Hand washing is the most effective method of decreasing the chance of catching colds and flu. You may wish to carry hand gel with you for occasions when washing is not convenient.
- Also, take extra care with cuts and scrapes: cleanse them thoroughly, use an antiseptic, and apply sterile dressings. Bring to the attention of your doctor any infection that is worsening.
- Chest infections may worsen quickly and become pneumonia. If you have such an infection, tell your doctor right away.

What should I do if I get a temperature?

Unless your doctor has advised you otherwise:

- Take paracetamol as directed on the packet. (Don't take anything containing aspirin because this can aggravate bleeding or bruising problems.)
- Drink plenty of fluids (water, tea, coffee, soft drinks).
- If the high temperature persists, or you start to feel worse, consult your doctor.

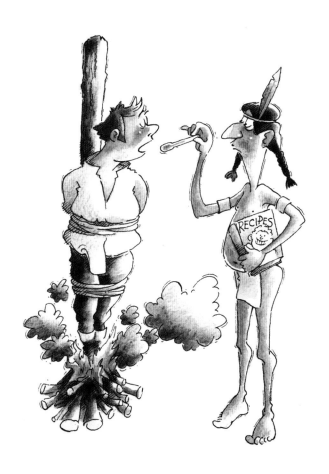

What if my MDS progresses to leukaemia?

MDS is a group of diseases that have many differences. It is important to diagnose the type of MDS to make the best treatment choices. With some types of MDS, a person may live with few symptoms for years, while other types can be life-threatening within months. In addition, some types of MDS are more likely than others to develop into acute myelogenous leukaemia (AML). See *Risk Scores* on page 31 for more information.

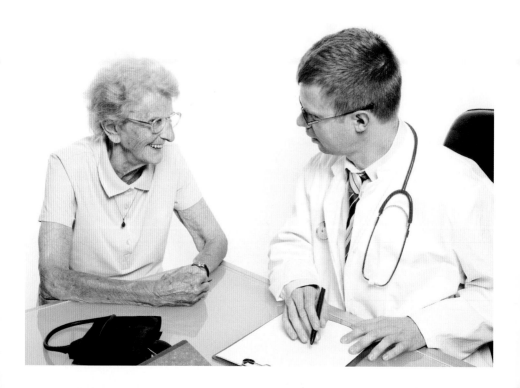

What are the aims of treatment?

The main aim of treatment in MDS is to get the number and type of blood cells in circulation back to normal. In the long term this may be done with a bone marrow transplant (see page 26) or with drug treatments (pages 27 and 28). In the short term a good way of boosting the blood cell count is by a transfusion – either with whole blood or with a blood extract, depending on what is needed. Transfusions may be used alone or in combination with other treatments.

I have heard that blood transfusions can be dangerous

Will I be carefully monitored if I have transfusions?

● Many people with MDS need blood transfusions to manage symptoms caused by low numbers of red blood cells and/or platelets. All donated blood is checked for any possible infections. The risk of infection from a transfusion in Europe is therefore very small.

● Red blood cell transfusions reduce problems with being very tired and short of breath.

● Platelet transfusions reduce risks of bleeding problems caused by very low numbers of platelets.

If you have MDS, your doctor will determine when you need transfusions and manage the possible risks. To manage transfusion risks, your doctor may:

● Give you additional treatment to remove iron from the body (iron chelation therapy). After many red blood cell transfusions, iron builds up in the body, causing organ damage.

● Give as few platelet transfusions as possible to limit the risk of the immune system developing antibodies (immune cells) that attack transfused platelets. If this happens, platelet transfusions must be closely matched to the patient.

● Treat blood cells with radiation and filter out white blood cells before transfusion. This reduces the risks of an immune system reaction.

Are there other ways to increase haemoglobin levels?

A person with MDS may be given drugs known as growth factors which help the body make more blood cells and so reduce the need for red blood cell transfusions. However, in many cases of MDS, the bone marrow where new blood cells are formed does not respond to growth factors.

Growth factors may also be given after a bone marrow transplant. In this case, growth factors often are effective. They can help speed up new blood cell production, reducing a person's need for transfusions and risk of infection.

What are the long-term effects of repeated blood transfusions?

Repeated blood transfusion leads to iron overload. The consequence of this accumulation of iron can be damage to various organs, particularly the liver and heart. In some cases, there may be iron accumulation in bones and joints. Excessive iron can be removed from the body by drug treatment known as iron chelation therapy.

Deferriprone is an oral iron chelator which needs to be taken 3 times per day. It is effective in some situations. Patients' white blood cell counts have to be carefully monitored on a weekly basis. Some recent reports suggested that the combination of deferoxamine with deferriprone is more effective than either agent alone in removing iron from the heart.

Deferriprone and deferasirox differ also in terms of their pharmacodynamics and metabolism. Deferasirox is almost completely excreted in faeces, whereas deferriprone is excreted in the urine. Another advantage of deferasirox is that it is not toxic at the bone marrow level. This feature, in particular, makes it very promising for use in this disease.

There is a low occurrence of side-effects when chelation is used as approved by regulatory bodies in Europe. A burning sensation at the site of delivery into the vein is common. Rarer side-effects include fever, headache, nausea, stomach upset, vomiting, bone marrow depression (dropping blood cell counts), a drop in blood pressure, and lowered levels of calcium in the blood. Kidney toxicity is a safety concern, but a rare occurrence.

DID YOU KNOW?

Chelation agents started out with very a different purpose from their use in lowering iron levels. They were introduced into medicine as a result of the use of poison gas in World War I. The first widely used chelating agent, the organic dithiol compound dimercaprol (also named British Anti-Lewisite or BAL), was used as an antidote to the arsenic-based poison gas, Lewisite. The sulphur atoms in BAL's mercaptan groups strongly bond to the arsenic in Lewisite, forming a water-soluble compound that entered the bloodstream, allowing it to be removed from the body by the kidneys and liver. BAL had severe side-effects.

After World War II, a large number of navy personnel suffered from lead poisoning as a result of their jobs repainting the hulls of ships. The medical use of EDTA as a lead chelating agent was introduced. Unlike BAL, it is a synthetic amino acid and contains no mercaptans. EDTA side-effects were not considered as severe as BAL.

In the 1960s, BAL was modified into DMSA, a related dithiol with far fewer side effects. DMSA quickly replaced both BAL and EDTA, becoming the US standard of care for the treatment of lead, arsenic, and mercury poisoning, which it remains today.

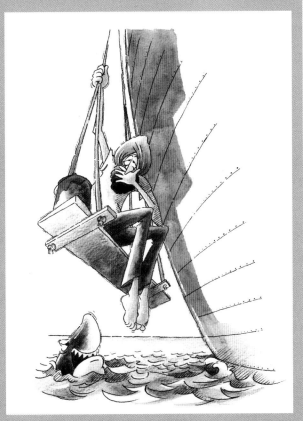

Does bruising have an effect on my health?

Bruising is simply blood leaking out of the blood vessels into the surrounding skin and muscle. MDS can lower the number of platelets in the blood which help control bleeding (these clump together and block small holes in the blood vessels). You will tend to bruise more easily but this is generally not a serious concern. Even so you should be more careful about everyday knocks and bumps, even people holding your arms or hands too tightly. A severe bruise can turn into an ulcer so you need to check with your doctor particularly if they happen on your lower legs.

Small injuries may become worse because of MDS. If you notice spontaneous bleeding, perhaps from your nose or when brushing your teeth, unusually heavy bleeding from small wounds, or perhaps from your bowels, urinary system, or vagina, contact your doctor right away.

MYTH

Black eyes (blood tracking down from a bruise on the forehead or eyes) can be treated successfully by pressing raw steak on to them.

Possibly true, but it has more to do with the massaging and movement of the blood within the bruising than anything else. Tends to tenderise the meat as well!

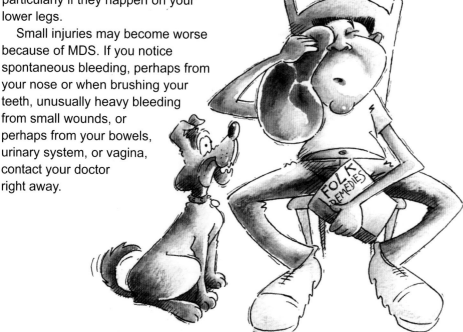

Am I suitable for a bone marrow transplant?

A bone marrow transplant (also known as a stem cell transplant) replaces the abnormal cells in the bone marrow with healthy blood-forming cells (stem cells). If a transplant may be a treatment option for you, your doctor will refer you to a transplant doctor for a consultation.

Doctors use certain factors to decide whether a person is suitable for transplant. It is not all clear-cut but revolves around certain clinical risks. Referral for possible transplant is recommended for patients with an intermediate-2 or high risk score who have one or more of the following factors:

- More than 5% blasts (the undeveloped cells) in the bone marrow.

- Intermediate or high-risk cytogenetic factors.

- Low blood counts for more than one type of blood cell (red blood cells, white blood cells and platelets).

A transplant doctor can also help determine the best time for a transplant. An early consultation with a transplant doctor enables your doctors to plan ahead even if a transplant is not your first treatment choice. The transplant doctor can begin the search for a suitable donor among family members or donor registry.

A transplant can offer some people the chance for a long-term remission of disease and a longer life, but it is not an option for all patients. A transplant may be a good option for people who have a suitable donor or cord blood unit and are healthy enough to tolerate a transplant. In general, younger patients tend to do better after a transplant than older patients. However, advances in transplant have enabled more older patients to undergo a transplant successfully.

Transplants

Allogeneic transplant

The standard transplant for MDS is allogeneic, which uses blood-forming cells from a family member, an unrelated donor or a cord blood unit (blood from the umbilical cord which has less chance of rejection if there is no other transplant option). The donor for a transplant must closely match the patient's tissue type. The best donor is usually a brother or sister with matching tissue type.

Reduced-intensity transplant

Before a transplant, a patient receives high-dose chemotherapy with or without radiation therapy. Many patients with MDS are older and have other health problems that may make them unable to tolerate this high-dose treatment. However, some may be able to tolerate a reduced-intensity treatment, which uses lower doses of chemotherapy and low-dose or no radiation therapy.

Reduced-intensity transplant is a newer approach to transplant for MDS, and early results have been encouraging. The use of reduced-intensity transplant to treat MDS is growing. This approach may offer the chance for long-term survival to some patients, especially those who are older or have other health problems.

Autologous transplant

As already noted, the standard transplant for MDS is allogeneic, which uses blood-forming cells from a family member, an unrelated donor or a cord blood unit. Another type of transplant is an autologous transplant, which uses the patient's own blood-forming cells. An autologous transplant is a standard treatment for some diseases and is being studied in clinical trials as a treatment for MDS. An autologous transplant may be an option for patients who do not have a suitable donor for an allogeneic transplant.

In an autologous transplant, blood-forming cells are collected from the patient. The patient is treated with high-dose chemotherapy and possibly radiation therapy, and then receives his or her own cells back.

A patient has higher risks of a relapse of MDS after an autologous transplant. This may be because disease cells can be returned to the patient along with his or her blood-forming cells.

Chemotherapy

Chemotherapy uses drugs to destroy abnormal cells or stop them from growing sometimes followed by a transplant. A treatment option for some people with severe MDS may be induction chemotherapy. Induction chemotherapy is very intense. The goal is to bring the disease into remission (no more signs of disease).

Induction chemotherapy may be an option for patients with high IPSS risk scores who are in good overall health but do not have a suitable donor for a transplant. Induction chemotherapy is also sometimes used to bring MDS into remission before a patient receives a transplant.

About half of patients treated with induction chemotherapy may reach a remission, but relapse is common and the rate of long-term survival is low, particularly in older patients. Because of the high relapse rate, patients may be given further treatment, such as a transplant or more chemotherapy.

In addition, many people with MDS, especially those who are older or who have other health problems, may be unable to tolerate intensive induction chemotherapy. Different chemotherapy treatments for MDS, some low-intensity and some high-intensity, are being studied in clinical trials to try to find a more effective approach.

When chemotherapy is taken by mouth or injected into a vein or muscle, the drugs enter the bloodstream and can reach cancer cells throughout the body (systemic chemotherapy). The way the chemotherapy is given depends on the disease being treated.

Much research is being done to find better treatment options for patients with MDS. Many newer drug therapies have been shown to bring a response. In some patients with MDS the goal is a long-term remission of the disease and long-term survival. For many other drug therapies, the goal is to improve a person's blood counts and symptoms. Managing the symptoms and related problems of MDS may offer a higher quality of life and a somewhat longer life than supportive care alone.

If you have MDS, talk with your doctor about the many newer drug therapies available (see page 28). Your doctor can help you determine which, if any, are good options for you. Your doctor can also help you find clinical trials offering these treatments, if they are appropriate for you.

Drug therapies when a transplant is not possible

Unfortunately, not everyone with MDS will be able to have a marrow transplant but treatment is still possible and can significantly improve their life. There are a limited number of therapies available. Azacitidine (also known as Vidaza) is a cancer medication that, while not being a cure for MDS, interferes with the growth of cancer cells, helping some mechanisms of the cells that keep growth under control to function properly, ultimately slowing their growth.

How is the drug given?

There is no form of the medicine you can take by mouth so it is given as an injection, usually by a health professional.

You may also be given medications to reduce nausea and vomiting while you are receiving treatment.

This medication is usually given for 7 days in a row every 4 weeks for at least 6 treatment cycles. But it all depends on the individual and their response to the treatment.

Unfortunately the drug can lower the blood cells that help your body fight infections. This can make it easier for you to bleed from an injury or get sick from being around others who are ill. To be sure your blood cells do not get too low, your blood will need to be tested on a regular basis. Contact your doctor at once if you develop signs of infection.

Other drugs

● Antithymocyte globulin (ATG) may be used to lessen the need for transfusions in patients with a certain form of myelodysplastic syndrome.

Where can I get more information?

Your doctor or pharmacist can provide more information.

Meeting a stealth disease

Some years ago I was getting more and more tired, with no energy even for everyday tasks. I had a health check and the blood test showed a serious lack of haemoglobin. Follow-up consultations, including an introduction to bone marrow biopsy, revealed an MDS condition.

A regime of blood transfusions began. It takes about two hours to absorb a unit of blood. Three units occupy the best part of a whole day and it seemed no time before I needed three units of blood every three weeks.

Sure, the transfusions did the trick in restoring some vitality in life, but the process of sitting in a hospital ward for a whole day became more and more tedious. And that's not all: very soon, the ferritin levels in my blood exceeded the 1,000 mark and I needed iron chelation therapy, which is far more uncomfortable and intrusive than transfusions.

Then, a breakthrough. I was enrolled on a clinical trial of a new medication having proven efficacy in the USA where it had been in use for a year or two.

The results were spectacular. In little time, haemoglobin levels had risen, without the need for further blood transfusions. As dependence on outside supplements of blood diminished, so did the need for iron overload chelation.

The clinical trial lasted for a year. That was two years ago, since when I have required neither blood nor iron chelation.

What the future holds is of course uncertain. I'll be 80 next year, so why should I care? Now, I live with a quality of life I could not even have imagined in the dark days of blood transfusions and iron chelation.

Mine is a relatively mild form of MDS. Other patients with more severe types of the disease will be suffering far worse symptoms than I ever did. New medication exists for these higher risk forms of MDS.

Am I getting the best treatment for my MDS?

There is often a broad range of options for treatment depending on the state of the condition in each individual patient. It can be difficult for someone to know how well the treatment is going, not least because the response is so variable. People with the same risk score and type of MDS can still respond differently to treatment. A person's age, overall health and other factors all influence his or her response to the disease and treatment. A doctor will also look at all these factors when planning treatment. If you have MDS, it is important to talk with your doctor about what type of MDS you have and your risk score. Ask how this information affects your treatment options.

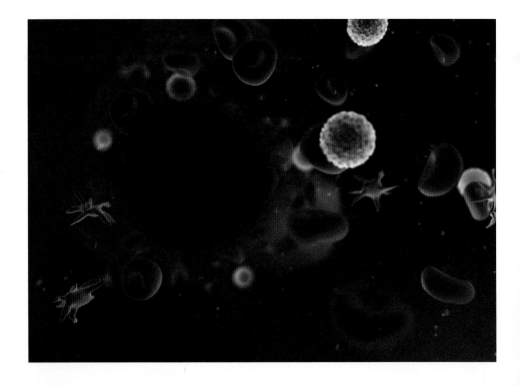

RISK SCORES

Although the type of MDS can help predict the course of a person's disease, people with the same type of MDS may respond to the disease and to treatment differently.

To try to better predict people's outcomes, researchers have developed several systems for defining types of MDS. The earliest is the FAB classification (from **F**rench, **A**merican and **B**ritish researchers). This takes account of several different disease factors, including the percentage of blasts in the bone marrow, to define five types of MDS. The later World Health Organisation (WHO) system is similar but divides MDS into eight types.

MDS risk scores

Researchers have developed another system for classifying MDS. This system is called the international prognostic scoring system (IPSS). The IPSS risk score describes the risk that a person's disease will develop into AML or become life-threatening.

A doctor may use the IPSS risk score along with the MDS type (see page 4) to plan treatment. The IPSS risk score is based on three factors that have been shown to affect a patient's prognosis:

● The percent of cells in the bone marrow that are blasts.

● Whether one, two or all three types of blood cells are low (also called cytopenias). The three types are red blood cells, white blood cells and platelets.

● Changes in the chromosomes of bone marrow blood cells. This may be called cytogenetics (the study of chromosome abnormalities). It may also be called the karyotype (a picture of the chromosomes that shows whether they are abnormal).

A person may have an IPSS risk score of low, intermediate-1, intermediate-2 or high risk. Doctors can use the risk score to plan treatment. Someone with low-risk disease may be likely to survive for years with few symptoms. That person may need less intense treatment. Someone with intermediate-1, intermediate-2 or high-risk disease may be likely to survive only if he or she receives aggressive treatment, such as a transplant.

Supportive care

What does it mean?

Supportive care will be part of the treatment plan for all people with MDS. The goal of supportive care is to manage disease symptoms and related problems.

For some people, supportive care may be the only treatment needed. Some people with few symptoms may need only regular doctor visits. The doctor will watch for any signs that the disease is getting more severe.

Some people with severe MDS may also choose supportive care as their only treatment. People who are older or who have other health problems may be unable to tolerate stronger treatment. Other people weigh the possible risks and benefits of different treatment options and choose supportive care. Supportive care does not offer the possibility of a long-term remission from MDS, but it may offer a way to manage a person's symptoms. Supportive care includes:

Transfusion therapy

- Transfusion therapy (blood transfusion) is a method of giving red blood cells, white blood cells, or platelets to replace blood cells destroyed by disease or treatment.

Patients who receive frequent red blood cell transfusions may have their tissues and organs damaged from the build-up of extra iron. Iron chelation therapy is a treatment that uses drugs that attach to the extra iron. The drug and the iron are removed from the body in the urine.

- Deferoxamine may be used to treat the build-up of too much iron in the blood of patients receiving blood transfusions. It is sometimes given with vitamin C.

- Platelet transfusions are usually given when the patient is bleeding or is having a procedure that may cause bleeding.

Growth factor therapy

- Erythropoietin may be given to increase the number of red blood cells and lessen the effects of anaemia. Sometimes granulocyte colony-stimulating factor (G-CSF) is given with erythropoietin to help the treatment work better.

Antibiotics

- Antibiotics may be given to fight infections.